DAWN AFTER DARKNESS

Rohit Gupta

Invincible Publishers

First published in India in 2018

ISBN: 978-93-87328-70-9

Invincible Publishers

G-120, Sushant Lok III, Sector 57, Gurgaon-122002

Registered Address: Opposite Kasturba Ashram, Radaur, Haryana - 135133

Printed at Thomson Press (India) LTD

Testimonials

It was about four years ago that Rohit came to my Foundation, IHIF and told us his story. Rebuilding his life, going through the pain and agony of physical therapy and the distressingly slow pace of neuro-rehabilitation, he has been through it all. Deserted by most friends and many family members, he has faced depression, trauma and loneliness through the recovery process. But Rohit not one to give up easily, has rebuilt his life, come out on top and is today facing the environment much better than most of us around him. Dawn after Darkness is an inspiring Saga of bravery and recovery. A must read for all TBI victims, caregivers and indeed all of humanity.

- Maharaja Gajsingh of Jodhpur, Chairman Indian Head Injury Foundation

"Dawn after Darkness" is the story of a young man in the prime of his life, whose existence went through a tumultuous roller coaster ride as he fell from the second floor of a hotel. Rohit's recovery from a TBI against all odds "Hits the reader in the head as well as the Heart"; and whether you are recovering from a TBI or supporting someone with it, this book will encourage you on your journey of healing, hope and meeting everyday challenges. After reading the manuscript, I believe that people like Rohit are the real heroes and brave men of this world.

- Commodore Ranbir Talwar, Executive Director, Indian head Injury Foundation

A Brain Injury can change one's life in a flash. Rohit has gone through it all and has come out with his story "Dawn after Darkness" which is a chronicle of immense courage and tenacity which was essential to bring him out of the Dark phase and face the world on his own terms. He has been a regular at the IHIF Rehabilitation Centre in Delhi and we have seen him making slow but sure progress towards independence. His book is exceptional in bringing out the pain and agony of a TBI victim and the suffering one faces from human apathy.

- Dr. Rajendra Prasad, Senior Consultant, Neurosurgery & Spine Surgery Indraprastha Apollo Hospitals, New Delhi & Hon. Medical Director, Indian Head Injury Foundation

Acknowledgement

Zero awareness and panic can lead us into an abyss. Finding the initial source of support through family was a blessing and ultimately, learning to swallow the bitter truth of TBI was a bigger blessing. I can never thank my family enough for their endless support. I would also like to extend my thanks to Indian Head Injury Foundation (IHIF), which is headed by Mr. Ranbir Talwar (Director, Delhi). It was because of his and his team's efforts that I was able to find a good rehabilitation centre that headed me to an efficient team of therapists and conducive machinery, contributing to my growth in every aspect. Further, I want to thank all my attendants and doctors without whose guidance this journey wouldn't be complete.

The IHIF helped me grow my network and exposed me to a world where I got an opportunity to meet many other TBI survivors, brain injury experts and those who are willing to learn about TBI. The aim of the awareness walks and programs organized by the IHIF wasn't limited to rehabilitation of affected one, but enlightenment of general public as it is them who ultimately suffer either as TBI survivors or family members of those who have been injured.

Moreover, the scope is not limited to head injury but it concerns all neurological disorders as well. It focuses not only on physical rehabilitation, but also mental which is necessary for growth and upliftment.

IHIF is an organization, established and funded by Maharaja of Jodhpur, his highness Maharaja Gaj Singh Ji after his son Yuvraj Shivraj Singh experienced the same devastating pain and injury during a polo match.

Contact details

Website: www.indianheadinjuryfoundation.org

Facebook: https://www.facebook.com/IHIFNRG/

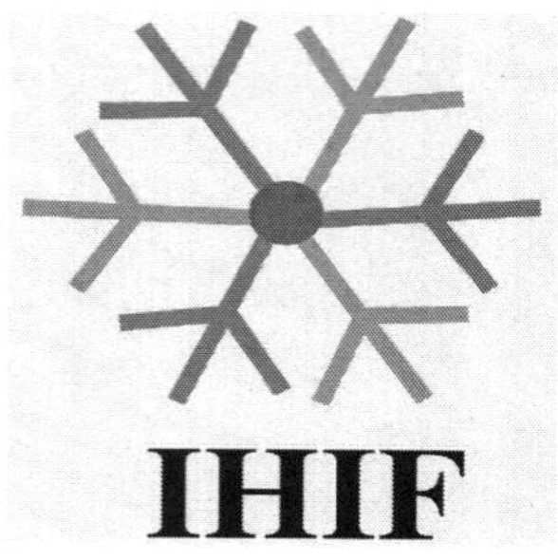

Introduction

Traumatic brain injury (TBI) is an invisible injury. It affects the operating system of the body which controls every bodily function. With a faulty operating system the whole body suffers, your heart mourns, and everything requires constant repairing. In India, especially, it's really difficult to explain brain injury as no one understands it. When you get moving, people begin torturing you with an inquisitive and overfriendly nature, inflicting pain.

TBI is not something which can be healed just by medicine and rest. The healing process is like a cross-country race, testing your patience, endurance, and most importantly your tranquillity. It takes quite some time and lots of hard work and continuous repetition. It requires physiotherapy, or exercise, to bring one back in shape, so you can move every body part without any restriction. It also requires speech therapy, for speech that has completely gone or is partially impaired, depending on the extent of the injury. It especially requires persistence.

Onlookers in India do not always understand the importance of continuing physiotherapy and speech therapy because the results are slow and perhaps not always visible. However, these therapies make a whole lot of difference, not just to the body, with its balance, posture, speech and fluency, but also to the personality.

After traumatic brain injury, things that used to be easy become much harder. You have to put in lots of effort for activities you have been doing all your life effortlessly. It becomes clear that life was much easier.

Traumatic brain injury is an injury which makes one realize the worth of life. It cannot be compared with any suffering, nor is it worth comparing, however, it is worth talking about, especially in India where there is zero awareness and tolerance regarding TBI and no one understands its complexity or severity.

It has been several years since my accident and despite the fact that I have overcome so many of my limitations, sometimes certain things remind me of that time and I return back to the worst phase of my life, the time I hated the most. I get very upset and feel useless.

I want to write about something else, other than Traumatic Brain Injury but whenever I begin to jot down my thoughts only Traumatic Brain Injury - my limitation, appears on the surface. Since, that's the root cause why I am lagging behind and have lack of self-confidence, I want people in general to know about it and treat normally those of us who have experienced it.

Traumatic brain injury can only be explained by a person who experiences it and by the care givers, as they know its true meaning and consequences that follow.

This is my story.

MY FIRST CRUSH

It was more ofa mischief that got my attention on her at a really tender age. Maybe, she has her own version regarding the same (describing as stupid cupid thing).

I would discuss it with my best friend rather than confronting myself and encouraging myself to go forward with my feelings. Inspired by Bollywood, tried catching her best friend's attention to get linked with her and teased, literally eroding my feelings.

I, my friend and she with her friend were seated on corresponding benches resulting in accentuating my feelings and flirting started. Cracking jokes and being the macho of the classroom, being accessible to her, obvious, isn't it?

Final semester exams for class IXth were approaching and the time to confront her finally arrived.

Card (Archie's) and some chocolates which I didn't offer immediately, as I was over-powered by excitement and enthusiasm.

It was the last exam, so let's go and celebrate and release all the stress. It was also the proposal day.

Beginning the celebration with lunch at Burger villa in Connaught place and post lunch I was all prepared to offer the card highlighting the same, very scared and intimidated with fear of refusal, so handled the card to my friend to approach her and ran a block away. Panting and curiously awaiting for a reply.

My friend approached me with a mischievous look, but a definite grin on his face. Hence, putting me in a state of confusion. So, he tells me her reaction and his method of flooding her with my feelings.

Brother, she was furious and spewing anger, but yes! She accepted your proposal.

Party was over, heading back home and exchanging phone numbers, but there's confusion on the girl's part.

INCEPTION

Like they say the beginning is hardest, this wasn't any different in this case.

Being a bully and mischievous was known for all wrong reasons.

For a first few days there was a gossip spread that a sweet girl was dating someone of contrary nature, even few approached to not get into this.

Being adamant will surely convince her, work things out and by making her BFF's word not worthy, yes, it did take some time on her part to sort things out in her mind before getting into commitment. Majority of the time went convincing her and making her believe that will be serious in this. Her BFFwas saying the contrary and putting words in her mouth.

It looked really worth then (time and energy spent).

We talked over phone (landline) not for long hours though and I was even scolded by her father, when my sister stepped in, transferring blame on her (wow, I love my sister).

Those were early days in our relationship and excitement was mounting on, especially for me.

As it was class 10th, pressure of studies was evident on her face, but I apparently kept her occupied in talks. Yes, she was interested but certain insecurities kept her on the edge, not avoiding but insecurity secluded her, many times.

Many relationships were budding then and influenced by them I skipped the bus ride in afternoon and made her skip hers as well. Both would share an auto (public transport) and would drop her and take another ride thereon or metro. We also found a spot near metro (place to hang in) which was least 'Bansals' crowded, hence safe.

No worries about future, just living the moment. The future plans were processing, regards amateur love.

Metro pillars were also a shed for seeing off before another day of school.

There were so much love and regular meetings, but we did not ignore examinations, preparation and tuitions since we got to spend time during school hours and our auto rides back home, which brought us, more close in every way.

E & G

Two specified classroom sections of commerce with math, separated but parallel classrooms, had same vicinity and close proximity.

It was a big break for every student, being promoted to class 11th and relive after what everyone had thought was the most pressurised situation and time.

It was a crucial time of our lives continuing with an unfaithful love story.

School bunks and a kindling love story. School bunks were a major part of class 11th minus attending school (which was also fun sometimes) enduring which the relationships went to another level; the love, the physicality, the feelings and most importantly attention.

School trips

The first school trip, in the first session of class 11th included almost everyone from all streams.

It was exciting, especially the excitement of travelling with that one special person. Since I and she didn't share the same classroom, missing on classroom intimacy was now being cherished. On reaching our destination, Manali, we checked into our hotel where the girls and boys room were in close proximity, but the teachers' room was quite not far .either.

I remember sneaking into the girls' room at midnight to meet her and on hearing loud squeak (her voice was like that) of our teacher, I used to go hide at the edge of the balcony. Fun fact: a friend used to imitate her.

All the boys will get drunk at night and act in a funny way.

There were some good conversation, promises anda little romance during the bus ride.

CLASS XIIth

A different floor, adjacent class room and more seriousnessas the final and most crucial year of school was commencing.

The start of the year was bitter as few good friends had flunked the previous year, the essence of the journey through class XIth.

Continuing, it was a year of group tuitions, future planning and also, a year of parties.

Two states

It was an indication, but being overpowered with love and pretentions of separation, signs from God was taken lightly.

She was shifting to a different city, and we were convinced that we can manage a long distance relationship. We even changed our numbers for free long distance calls.

Although, it was going good but long distance has a negative impact. I used to make several trips to visit her without informing my relatives residing in the same city.

Years passed, rather comfortably, but the doom day awaited us.

Thought of fear of future never crossed my mind and I was all prepared for the most awaited trip of a youngster's life, GOA.

The trip turned out to be a disaster for me and my family. Still living and coping with the injury for a better future, which taught me important lessons.

THE END

It was decided by destiny. Way things were preceding, it was proclaimed much earlier than the actual confrontation but the same was shocking and unbelievable as circumstances demanded empathy. Sympathy would have been offending, from someone so close. Disposing off the relationship like scrap was agonizing initially, but the fight ahead was of much more importance because of the broken present. Breaking all ties over messenger was something that made me believe "only, family sticks around during thick and thin".

Accepting the new was burdening enough, accompanied with betrayal.

Chapter One

Life Before, And the Injury

I led a normal life like many other kids for my first 20 years. I was just a conventional kid raised in a Delhi suburb. I went to school, made friends, got punished, bunked school and hung out with friends.

The first major challenge of life was when my parents sent me to a hostel in Class 8th. I experienced living life on my own without family comfort and managed almost everything on my own, like my dirty laundry, my homework (which was a big task) and many other things. I was also ragged on by the seniors, until I unleashed a side of me which they called as 'the original Delhi bully', and nicknamed 'gunda'.

While life felt normal, there was something that was different about me. It felt like everyone else was alike, and I was the one who kept getting pointed out. It took me a while to notice it. Also, I was always known as the most mischievous child of the family, even though others were also a part of our mischief setup.

Recalling old memories of myself, as a young adult, I realize now that I definitely had Attention Deficit Hyperactivity Disorder (ADHD). I was a hyperactive kid who constantly sought the attention of everyone around me. Hyperactivity helped in keeping me fit, and it made me entertaining and charming, but it also landed me in big trouble.

The second major challenge of my life was being thrown out of the hostel. Mr. T.W. Philips, my then principal, noticed my nature in just nine months. I had terrible grades in eighth class. He saw that I was a hyperactive, restless and troublesome kid and he knew I would get in deep trouble and worsen things for myself and my family. If I had paid attention then, things would have been better now.

My dad somehow managed to get me back in my old school, where after passing Class 9th, I met a girl who became a special friend. In Class 10th, I was anxious, as in Delhi we have CBSE board exams that help determine your subjects for senior-secondary examinations, and thus your career. When I passed the exams, it was like a victory!

After that, I relaxed a little. Class 11th was like a break, bunking school, going on vacations with friends and roaming around playing snooker. It was all about having fun before the ultimate test which was Class 12th. Up to this time, life had been simple and quite easy. I passed this final year with what I considered good marks but the competition outside was very tough. I was awarded admission in a college based on my marks but in the end I sat for a university entrance examination and was given admission through a management quota in a professional college where I began pursuing law.

Once college life started, my school friends, except for two, drifted away and my special friend went to another state. However, I made many new friends in college and we had fun. Even exams ended up being fun, because of the group study. My friends called me 'baniya' and life was all about living it up, with no worries at all. In Hindi, I would say 'zindagi umda thi.'

Seven years after those first words of warning from my principal, Mr T.W. Philips, on Tuesday 6 April, 2011, I hit the third challenge of my life.

Of course, I had no idea it was coming and everything seemed entirely normal leading up to that day.

On Sunday 20th March, 2011, it was Holi. Many of my friends came to my place to celebrate the festival of colours, drinking 'bhang' and partying together. We pretended to be sober but our inebriation showed in our actions and on our faces.

On March 30, 2011, India played Pakistan in the cricket World Cup semi-finals. I and three of my friends who went to watch the match, at Mohali, cheering madly for India who won the match, taking one step closer to the World Cup. The next Thursday, 2nd April, was a huge day in India's history: the World Cup final was being played in Mumbai. Unfortunately my parents didn't allow me to go to Mumbai along with my friends, but when India won the World Cup after 28 years, I and my friends partied all night anyway, singing and shouting.

As compensation for not being allowed to go to Mumbai for the finals, my parents let me go to Goa on Monday 4th April, 2011, with a few friends and my special friend. We reached Goa on Tuesday 5th April and checked into a second floor room of a Resort Hotel named Winsor-Bay.

That night was the last crazy party of my life.

We rented motorbikes, like everyone does in Goa, and all went clubbing and drinking. I danced and sang songs and had a great time. We all returned to our Hotel to our room around 3 am. After some nasty stuff, I went outside to get some air on the balcony. The parapet looked to me like a good place to sit to relax, so I began to climb up.

After that, I don't remember anything.

***

Six months later, I woke up.

I opened my eyes and saw my immediate family around me. "Ooo...waaa, waa." Noises came out of my mouth like squeaks. I couldn't speak, and I hardly understood what was going on around me.

"What happened?" I managed to communicate with my mother at some point later.

"You were in Goa, with your friends," she said. "You had a bike accident, and now you have a head injury."

"Wasn't I wearing a helmet?"

"You were," she said. She looked away. "But the impact was too strong."

But I was curious. A bike accident? How did it happen? And why did I remember being out on the balcony? It wasn't until later that a friend told me what he knew.

Yes, I had been out on the balcony, and yes, I had probably climbed onto the parapet. That was probably how I fell off the balcony, landing on the hard cement ground, two storeys down.

I lay there for two hours, my mother said, until the hotel guard saw me. There was a mix-up with my motor-bike as well: by mistake I had brought the wrong bike back to the hotel with me after the club, and somehow the guys who had rented that bike turned up to claim it.

They ended up waking up my friends to tell them that I wasn't where they thought I was, and I was then hurried to a government hospital for first aid with the help of the hotel authorities and police.

Around 9 am on Wednesday 6th, my friend called my sister to tell her what had happened. She was at home, on leave from her office as she was preparing for her MBA exams.

"Rohit has met with a severe accident," my friend told my sister, "A head injury."

My sister immediately ran to our parents and told them the news. It was the third navratri, my parents left everything immediately and boarded the first flight to Goa. On the way they informed my cousins in Mumbai who also rushed to Goa and shifted me to a well-equipped hospital, the Apollo.

I was comatosed for six months. I could breathe on my own, but had a feeding tube down in my stomach. For the first month we stayed in Goa: after that my parents managed to get me back to Ganga Ram Hospital in Delhi using an Air Ambulance, where I stayed for another month. After that, they brought all the medical equipment I needed to our house, and I lay there for another four months, unconscious and comatose.

***

I had to learn everything all over again.

My speech was completely gone. The guy who was the most talkative person in our family couldn't speak. Learning to talk again was the most burdensome quarrelsome task for me. I knew everything that was going on around me, and I had all my faculties, but I just wasn't able to say anything.

Finding that I'd lost my speech was just the beginning though. Soon after I woke up, I tried to lift myself up from the bed. I failed. I felt generally weak, but I also had no strength in my limbs.

A few days passed and I was moving around in a wheel chair and communicating via notes, writing whatever I could in my phone. I had gained some strength as I started eating with my mouth and finally the artificial food pipe was removed from my stomach.

***

SEIZURES

Uncontrollable, unsettled and soul shrieking movement of body organs puts us in great horror. A few minor ones, when comatose, prepared my mother on how to handle such situations. For the first time post swallowing the bitter truth of TBI and after gaining partial consciousness, had one more severe seizure attack left every family member in a state of severe panic. The immediate step was to consult the neurosurgeon, since none had any answer to what had just occurred. I, the victim of all this adversity, felt more helpless in my partly conscious state before the beginning of a new life full of challenges beyond my imagination. The neurosurgeon advised my guardians to increase the dosage of my medication to stabilize and prevent the seizures and control the brain neurons which were barbarous/self-governing after this metaphorical re-birth. Months passed rather comfortably while I was busy governing and re-learning every body movement and speech, but was never able to digest the moment of shock and adversity. Moths later, we held a small gathering to celebrate my parents' anniversary and my complete consciousness, but my brain was prepared to give us another moment of shock and embarrassment. Everyone was curiously awaiting the cake cutting ceremony when another seizure hit me. The wheel-chair was on the verge of collapsing and hitting the ground when my mother's eye caught me, since all her attention was always focused on me despite whatever was happening around. My father ran to get hold of me, while my mother held me by my shoulders and transferred me to a bed. Remembering that one moment precisely sends chills down my spine, as my hands, feet and face had turned into that of a disfigured person. This time, we visited the neurosurgeon for a valid explanation, and he suggested changing my medication to a stronger one to control the brain neurons, since such seizures could be fatal. The new medication took time to settle, resulting in more sleep, but it had a better control over my brain. It helped focus on a full-fledged recovery, despite my apprehensions regarding the future, which were hidden as was confined to the walls of my home.

Soon we began speech therapy and first thing I thought was, 'How am I going to control my drooling?' I was dribbling like an infant, making my shirt wet. It was something I had never thought about before, controlling my saliva. I had also never, in my whole life, focused on how I speak. I'd never thought about my posture. For me, like for the vast majority of other kids, all these came with my first breath. Until I was on the other side of it, I hadn't remembered meeting even one person who had to focus on the way they talked or whether their body was properly aligned.

Five months after becoming partly conscious, I had no explanation for the things happening around me. I was unaware of why I was in such a helpless condition and why all these tubes were passing through me until I was given a valid explanation.

Being unable to speak a single word was the first sign of being totally dependent on others. I was communicating via messages and when I found out I couldn't walk either, I was transferred from one mode of dependency to another. After another six months of being in a wheel chair, I realized I was not the same person anymore. I had to emerge as a new personality. Still communicating via text messages, I started speech therapy and physiotherapy. Therapy sessions were my breakfast and lunch.

As time passed I gained strength and balance, and I started going out for walks with a servant in the park. That was hard enough. But the social awkwardness was harder. Every individual who passed stared at me, as though I had committed some heinous crime. They would come up to me to offer sympathy, hold my hand and try to help me.

"Oh, did you have a stroke, poor boy?"

"Poor child. You have a paralysis."

Some of them looked at me as if I was mentally unstable. Would I jump out at them or yell at them? They stared and stared.

Sometimes I got so frustrated. Should I answer them back, I wondered. Or frown at them? Perhaps I should stop going for walks. But it seemed ridiculous that I should have to delay my progress in recovery because of worthless, rude people who actually had no interest in me or my life, so finally I started ignoring them to their face.

My mother was doing every possible research about what could help me and enhance my recovery. She was always searching for something different, and one day, she took me to 'Hydro Therapy' which was very beneficial and fun at the same time. But whoever said that the world is full of alike people said right. Even in a specific pool for therapy, people asked the same silly questions and said the same silly things.

Chapter Two

Rehabilitation

Life is strange. One mistake turns everything upside down and by the time we realize it, time has already gone and it's late.

After the consequential time of my accident, I am ready to share my story. It's especially important in India, where brain injury and stroke cases are becoming very common; however, people mistake them for paralysis and complete handicap. In India there is no proper rehabilitation to treat a person with traumatic brain injury, but everyone has an opinion; telling you what you should do, how you do it and pointing out mistakes.

Traumatic brain injury is the worst thing that can happen to anyone because one has to again learn all the basic things in life and everything essential for being happy and confident. Before this life-changing incident I was very careless and never actually understood the value of life but, now I understand it very well. I have a clear picture in my mind. I feel how every TBI survivor must feel, sick, ruined and defeated at times, but there is nothing much we can do about it except accepting the harsh reality.

All cases of TBI are different. But in every case, it's a long, tiring and never-ending journey towards the recovery. Progress is very slow and takes lots of effort on the part of the TBI survivor and his or her family. Yes, surviving a brain injury feels like a 'rebirth', but this time around you are born mature and have to work on every single body part individually, and for quite some time.

Today I can walk independently, but it took lots of work on my part, on the part of the therapists and most importantly on the part of my parents who have been my support system, to get me here, and there's still a long road ahead. My speech is still not normal. I still struggle to speak, and walk on difficult paths. I am still doing physiotherapy on a daily basis as there's scope for improvement.

I'm a fortunate person to have had all this help. The cost of all these therapies is too much for most. Normal people struggling with life on a day-to-day basis cannot afford such an expensive treatment. There must be proper rehabilitation centres with all the facilities so that a TBI survivor can recover and become completely fit to continue life.

There are more severe impacts of brain injury on a person's life. I personally know people who have been comatose for more than a year. They cannot walk or use their limbs. I request all to respect their life, as it is very crucial.

Normal life is full of challenges and obstacles, which require lots of thinking before execution. Since my injury, sometimes when I see people talking, walking or running so easily without any effort, I start wondering if earlier these things were really that easy? Or did I just never pay any attention?

These little things in life are important. They deserve our attention and concern because we never value things we get easily and without effort – just a 'human nature'. These are God-given and should be respected. When we are born, with time we start walking and speaking, but we never really know the effort we put into it. It just came naturally with time and there was no effort at all. Post-TBI, living life is not impossible but it is challenging. When things get affected it takes lot of effort and sweat to fix them.

Today I feel disabled when I walk and talk because I cannot handle those questioning eyes staring at me, when

I try to look normal. Saying 'it does not matter' would be a lie. It does matter. It makes me self-conscious. I lose my confidence and patience and these periods are like avalanches in my recovery. I feel ashamed when I speak as I cannot match the speed of the person with whom I am conversing. I am not as clear as they are. Sometimes I mumble and chew my words because of such agonizing looks. I try my best to look normal, but I fail. Maybe the extra effort fails me, or maybe sometimes I feel like taking a break from everything, but when I do I feel guilty and as though I am delaying my recovery. I stumble and fall many times but whenever this happens I motivate myself by thinking, 'Well, at least I can walk. This is better than when I was unconscious.' And an inspiring quote "whenever you stumble, make it a part of the dance".

Recovering from brain injury is a long, tiring and stressful journey but one has to stay self-motivated. One cannot give up after reaching far. I have to finish this exceptionally overwhelming journey and continue the climb. Now, I tell myself, I need not hurry, but I need to be there. I need not walk fast but I must take small and definite/accurate steps. I need not speak fast but I will speak correctly and make it meaningful. I have to make sure I keep moving forward and that nothing on the way discourages and disheartens me. There are times when I feel weak, scared, lonely and mad but these are symptoms of betterment – really! – and progress, which one needs to deal with in a positive way.

Keep moving forward because it's your journey. You have to travel it alone because during tough times only hard work pays off. People might stop noticing the progress you have made but you know how far you've come, so it doesn't matter if people appreciate it or not (or at least, that's the lie you need to tell yourself.) You know your goal and you have come far to achieve it, so you can't stop.

My observation is that, being physically fit is the most important thing in life. Nothing else matters more.

Many people will point out your mistakes but they won't step forward to correct them. You yourself are the only one who has to take the initiative to correct them. You also have to get through the times when you get exhausted and feel discouraged at slow progress. This can be the time when you lose patience and start hating yourself, everything and everyone around you.

Recovering from TBI is complex and confusing. There simply isn't enough time in a day to do what you want to do, because the 'normal things' in life that help you recover take so long. I want to learn more to complete my education but when I take time to do that, I feel guilty of not doing my regular exercises and delaying my recovery. When I do my regular exercise I feel the opposite! In between I develop other interests like spreading awareness about Traumatic Brain Injury but I am quite confused about my interest in life, post-Traumatic Brain Injury.

Recovery is like evolution; one constantly experiences changes, and healing takes time with TBI. I might not be as 'good' as people expect, but I am recovering and gaining knowledge of things which were alienated from me in a fraction of a second. I haven't simply adapted to the situation or circumstances.

Brain injury is like sitting an exam for which you haven't prepared for. However, you have to finish it and pass with flying grades as there's no other option. Not only that, if you decide you will prepare for it, you soon realize that you cannot stop the preparation. You have to go on with it forever. It does not finish. The course is not limited. It is like an endless ocean that you must traverse.

Chapter Three

Speech

My speech is a big concern in my day-to-day life. It is something I have been stressing about since almost forever. Yes, I've seen some improvement, but for me 'improvement' is not enough. I can't settle for that. I'm not so concerned about how I walk (whether it's toe to heel or using my full foot). But my speech is different. It really is the biggest matter of concern for me, as it makes or breaks my day. I was never a slow talker before, but I had brakes and my enunciation wasn't bad. Now I slur my words due to hyper-salivation, and I'm fast! My words cross all the barricades and violate every rule.

I pledge to myself every day to take it slow but when the time comes, I race ahead and my tongue takes over. I get true pleasure and glory when I communicate exactly the way I sound in my mind – in other words, being precise. It gives me a sense of pride and joy within and I don't feel inferior to myself.

Mostly, I'm opposed to sympathy; I hate it, but my speech invites sympathy, and my fear of mispronouncing, stammering and repeating myself makes it worse. The hunger and desperation for betterment keeps me busy in my head. It feels like a nightmare that makes my eyes pop out. I cannot sit by and wait for my day and just hope everything will be good. Speech matters and correct enunciation helps in sailing smoothly.

In my mind, I remind myself over and over to be cautious while speaking. It's like flight attendants who tell passengers the safety tips when flying, even though when everyone knows about them. "Repetition, repetition and repetition". That's my speech story.

When I know what I'm trying to say and I've prepared, my fluency is not affected. It's much easier than speaking with one word per breath. However, one always doesn't have a prepared speech. I request and beg myself to 'please, speak slowly'. I must allow the air to be processed correctly, thus getting a good end result.

Sometimes it's hard to concentrate on my exercises and therapies due to my depression over my speech.

I'm often sad, gloomy and self-pitying, but anger is the biggest obstacle to good speech and so is depression. The former makes you blabber, and with the latter, you're lost in agony. But stressing too much doesn't help much, so at times, I've tried another approach – of being calm. Again, however, my impatience fails me.

I have all the words and phrases but being hyper and agitated disappoints me. Out of 24 hours in a day, during the time I am awake, I think about how to make my speech lucid. It may be that the extra effort, nervousness and over thinking minimises my charm.

I'm not yet tired, neither am I giving up. I'm not angry because I have to repeat myself constantly. I don't boil over when I get it wrong but, yes, I'm frustrated. I feel helpless when I'm not understood or am asked to text or write. I am repeating my words but I know the drill, please allow me to speak again for a little satisfaction.

If you are lacking proper speech, you are delayed in your responses, or you mumble, people doubt you. When my flawed speech is accompanied by my flawed balance, doubt about me increases. It is not only my fault. People are also to be blamed; they understand unimportant talk and behave deaf and dumb when the meaningful talk comes.

Words coming out of your mouth should be intelligible. Knowing that my speech creates obstacles and constantly lets me down, makes me feel I am doomed; I'm supposed to be content with what I have achieved to this date and cherish that, the rule book says. But it's not enough.

Half of the time I feel the confusion within as to whether I can satisfy the other person, but this leaves me unhappy and unsatisfied. My priority should be my betterment, which comes after communicating in a proper way. Being selfish isn't bad if it is propelling you and keeping you happy and motivated. Caring about the other person is good, but doing it at your own cost leaves you empty-handed and steals your happiness.

My self-confidence is at an all-time low because of my speech. It reflects badly on me, it scares me, and it keeps me on the back foot. My basic nature is to be convivial, this is how I've survived through my life but now my speech is an impediment to that.

Often, I hold back from speaking because I'm intimidated by the fear of getting it wrong or being looked upon as an intruder in a world of perfect people.

I have accepted that this speech issue might pester me for my whole life. There might not be any further improvements but that's not helping me either. My heart controls my mood, and my heart gets upset when people react badly to the way I speak. My life is a book of sad rhymes. I mourn every second, even after deciding to be happy and not to be bothered by anyone's comments.

Earlier, I felt angry due to my incompetence in balance and speech but in the following years, the vulnerability of not being able to communicate well made me even more susceptible to negativity. I really need patience if I'm going to have a better today. People looking on praise me for my bravery during hard times, and for becoming independent, but I'm still dependent! No one can understand me! The real hard work takes place now, as the current situation makes me vulnerable.

I have two options: either keep my mouth shut or walk my talk (one which the unconscious mind utters consciously). My speech spoils my image. I'm so near to being a good version of the 'new me' but the problems with my speech make me forget to appreciate anything I've achieved. Instead, I should rather focus on impressing myself.

I have learned things from posters, famous quotes and sayings by anonymous people: 'They say, it is better doing something than nothing,' and 'Seek first to understand... there will always be time later for judgment.'

People have no patience, and I include myself in that. I sometimes imagine myself in their shoes. I, too, would laugh, not pay much attention, and hurl insults, not knowing the reason behind someone's disability. It is really strange, how every person has an opinion and gives tips on how you can or should improve yourself. I listen if I respect the relationship or if the person giving advice is senior, but it seems odd that they don't realize that no-else would care for you more than you do, and you're probably trying everything that's under your control and within your limitations.

Looking at the other side of life, there are countless people facing severity in their respective lives, with situations I am unaware of. In such a situation shall I rejoice? I blush when I think that I am in a much better state than them. Perhaps, instead, should I regret my decisions? I know regretting now would make no difference nor it will reverse anything. Perhaps I should just try harder, and not give myself permission to sympathize with myself, feel disheartened, or sink deep in remorse. I have remorse about my reluctance to converse, my enunciation of words and phrases, and not living up to my own high expectations.

"It all takes time," people say. But that's not a rescue program from my viewpoint. I now know what the remedy is; it is 'not implementing it' that makes me sink in guilt – the guilt of failure, ignorance, being taken lightly, and inferior treatment. But I won't give up or give in to the current situation and will work hard for perfection.

Many are facing similar issues or worse but, thanks to the Lord, I have financial security and parents who understand my situation most of the time. The relationship we have is secure, but has been hampered and tested to every extent. We are all mature people who are dealing with something – TBI – that broke us. And the healing has been hard. We all try to control our emotions and are fortunate that at least we had each other when this storm hit us.

I know tricks that can back me up when I have a bad speech day but it's hard when every alternate day is a slap on the face. However, I believe that every morning is a fresh start and I will definitely speak in an organized manner and I shall continue to believe that, because I am capable of making it happen. I shall communicate in a language which makes enunciation complete and keeps me satisfied at the end of the day. Actually, I'm feeling good while enunciating and trying, not hesitating, and repeating. Also, by now I know the reactions because they are more predictable than me!

Chapter Four

Mood Swings

Traumatic Brain Injury can have the effect of making you short-tempered and impatient. For example, the things I am trying to say are very clear to me, but all too often, the other person doesn't understand at all and starts guessing, which irritates me and makes me angry. Almost daily I promise to do better, and scold myself to not shout and be patient, but eventually I break the promise.

Impatience also comes when I think I am the only one who is suffering with troubles in life. In the past I have ignored the problems, difficulties and challenges that others are facing, but this doesn't help those around me.

I may be fighting a 'fight' about which maybe no one knows, but I'm ignoring the fight my near and dear ones are fighting, in providing me with the best rehabilitation, and providing everything I need and demand. They silently bear all the nuisance and drama I create, without any complaint. I am doing all this work and therapy for myself but they are doing it for someone else - not out of any personal interest, but because they want to see their child independent and self-sufficient.

Every morning I get up with the motivation to settle unnecessary things popping in my head. I feel the pressure to ask, 'What is lacking? What am I doing wrong?' I'm motivated to do better, but then I, myself, spoil it because of my short temper. Every morning is charming and delightful but I fight unnecessarily with my parents, create a scene, and make it look ugly.

I very well know my speech is not clear. I have to speak slowly, putting emphasis on every word to be clear and make it sound presentable, but I shout at them for not understanding what I say. Short temper is the reason behind my delay in recovery and making improvements in my speech.

I feel I am sinking and going into depression because of my inability to communicate without effort. Every other normal human being can talk without exerting themselves. I am not affected by anything else - be it my posture, my walk or anything – it's my speech that is bringing me down and making me negative .

Frustrations multiply when dealing with Traumatic Brain Injury. You're uncertain about when and how you can get the desired results. I was always a short-tempered person, but brain injury has made me ill-tempered and infuriated. I have become a person who would scream and misbehave about everything said or done. I have disturbed the peace and created hatred in the environment and near me. I have shouted at people who built and shaped me; I have regretted it later, cursed myself and felt like running away. I might have overcome many disabilities and might look tough, but I am quite broken and shaken inside.

Frustration due to one's own incompetence is threatening, as it is a barrier in connecting with others. In many ways, frustration is equivalent to isolation. Instead of talking, we shout, and are not able to connect. Even the tiniest of creatures have a circle with whom they connect, even if it's just to hunt or attack. Humans are God's finest creation and we have ego which we use to connect with each other. Frustration leads to isolation because we terminate and disrupt our connections with anger and less communication. Isolation takes over quickly and makes you fearful, and yet you have to go out to find and know your limitations and fears.

What happened to me was a mistake; it wasn't destiny. Anger is a choice, not an escape, but frustration is an escape that creates hatred in your own heart and in the hearts of others as well, creating a barrier in bonding.

Dependency has an adverse effect on a person's personality, perhaps more than being handicapped. When you're handicapped you know you are dependent. When you're independent you think you might do something, but then create your own obstructions which create barriers.

It's frustrating when I do not see any visible changes in my progress, and I feel I have been sweating for nothing. (Of course, I forget sometimes that not all changes are visible to the naked eye.)

Frustration is depression, but it doesn't come with silence. Instead, it speaks with anger and screams in a squeaky voice. It's frustrating to be dependent on circumstances. You feel reluctant when you know you might just succeed.

I am still managing the frustration. It is teaching me a lesson; where to react, where not to, how to behave in every situation, and how to let things be.

Post TBI, it feels as if life is facetious and dependent on circumstances, and this changes my perspective on everything. I have to live life as it comes but being quiet and upset has become a habit. Mornings are encouraging and delightful but evenings are usually are depressing and take the life out of me.

Writing is good for releasing the tension and frustration and for expressing feelings in a way that does not harm anyone. I realized after my accident that penning down my thoughts and feelings gave me relief and a break from my debilitating thoughts.

Chapter Five

Friends and Family

When I woke up after six months of being comatose, I was shocked and surprised to see myself in such a disastrous state, with tubes passing through my body! I tried to ask my parents what happened but I couldn't speak so I asked with the help of actions which were not ambiguous.

"You went to Goa and met with a motorbike accident," they told me. "Discussing it isn't going to help."

There was no drama then. My parents narrated me the story of how it had apparently happened and told me that two of my friends had come all the way to Goa to visit me in the hospital, where I was fighting for my life. My parents' motivation helped me a lot to fight against Traumatic Brain Injury, and begin my recovery.

A year later after rigorous physiotherapy and speech therapy, and when I was at least fine enough to go out with my friends for hogging on road-side vans, one of my friends told me what actually happened.

"It wasn't a motorbike accident," he said. "Yes, you were in Goa. But you fell from the balcony on the second floor of the hotel."

I was stunned.

When I reached home, I discussed it with my parents.

"It's a shock," I said. "I've lived on the second floor all my life and never fallen off anything."

I was angry and upset, angry at my parents for not telling me the truth, and upset as I couldn't believe it. From the very next day I started working harder – perhaps more out of embarrassment than shock.

I no longer feel comfortable in the company of friends with whom I previously spent most of my time, not because they are faster than me in everything they do but because I find I have less in common with them. Over time they have grown and become more mature (they outgrew me), and have moved on.

My friends visited me often for the first two years but then the visits became abbreviated, seeing each other on birthdays, either mine or theirs. Today, years later, I don't see them often, and whenever I do meet them, I feel like a stranger. Half of the people about whom they talk I cannot relate to. I don't know the incidents that are being discussed as I have not been a part of them. I feel very estranged and keep asking questions. "When did this happen? Who did you people meet? Where did you go and what was the place like?"

I know I am not as fast as I used to be, but this doesn't mean everyone had to change their attitude towards me. Just because I cannot speak as fast and fluently as someone, doesn't mean that person should avoid me, or pretend to hear when they don't understand. I am trying my best to improve with every passing day but I can't beat time. I love my friends a lot but they need to understand me and my injury. I know people see me as a responsibility, rather than someone who can talk and contribute to the entertainment. I try to avoid help as much as I can and only ask for it when it's needed the most. I don't want sympathy - just normal treatment and the company of my friends.

I still want to be part of every conversation like before. I feel good when I get treated normally. Being a Gemini, I love extra attention but I don't want any kind of special treatment or sympathy. My friends have become strangers, known people have become unknown and my phone has become just a medium for stalking the outside world, so

I can keep myself up to date and know what is happening around me, not just news. We are not living in the 18th century, where phones and Internet were inaccessible. People could keep in touch if they wanted to. Long gone are the days when people use to say 'friends are forever and are always there for you'. Now it's just an old phrase. Earlier, I thought friends were for life, but now I have realized they have their own limitations and they cannot be there at all times. They support you initially but they are not present for the long and time consuming recovery after brain injury. You are alone, and you have to fight alone, which means finding a way to be happy, and doing something to keep yourself busy or your mind occupied.

It feels like life has come to a standstill, especially on weekends where life feels like a burden. You're stuck and want to move but then you realize you need company as you are not a tree! It's not necessary to have a gang of friends, sometimes just one person makes the difference to you feeling wanted and not alone. What I believed was out of love and friendship now feels like favour because of behavioural change and the time gap.

Sometimes I think about the past and ask myself, 'was I really that guy who was so outgoing and hardly used sit at home? Was I really such an extrovert?' I feel I have become a very confused person, and the exact opposite of what I was. Now, I think a lot before acting which is actually good; thinking before speaking, and speaking with a pre-determined mind gives good results, but it's not always possible.

I want to live despite my impediments, and fit into every situation. I wish to talk fluently and exchange my views with friends as an 'insider'. I don't know what they think or feel when I'm in their group but I feel like an outsider. I do not meet up with people so that I can feel I'm back in the hospital. I don't appreciate their 'favours' or sympathy or help. Their aim should be to make someone in my situation feel at home and comfortable, and not to alienate them just because they are different from how they used to be.

Their behaviour is what has pushed me away, and sometimes I want to share my anger and frustration with them.. However, when I've tried doing this with a few of them, I found they were no longer my friends.

My mother often says, "Go out meet your friends or they will forget you." As a matter of fact, they have forgotten me! I dodge her every time because I know the people she is talking about are no longer friends. They are just acquaintances who once thoroughly knew me, and vice-versa.

I feel that if I had skipped my short trip to Goa, I would be a totally different person today. However, if I think the other way around, I also could have met with an even more fatal accident. Maybe I would have died. There are various ways of looking at the same thing, and blaming someone else won't solve my problem; it might give me temporary relief but it will not put an end to my troubles. Only my own efforts against disability will bring a solution.

It has been tough to realize these harsh realities, but I also cannot ignore the fact that my friends literally picked me up from the pavement. I don't think it was a duty that made them do it. But it does make me ask, 'if they did it out of love, why have they forgotten me now?' And, if I have not been forgotten, why is there such disparity in the way they treat me?

Earlier, I assumed that being an extrovert was always an advantage to life, but now that I'm in circumstances that make me look unwanted, like I am looking for a place where I do not belong, it doesn't seem like an advantage any more.

There have been times where I have hated my friends. I have accepted the fact that friends are like clothes which wear out with time and are not suited to every situation. But there also were and are times where I am thankful for them and love them immensely. I blame myself for these changeable feelings, but my mind has become vulnerable to such despicable thoughts.

I am trying to start a new group of people who are in somewhat similar circumstances to me but they say it requires lots of effort to start something and attach people to it. Sometimes I feel frustrated and want to hit out at them. When I realize their feelings, I stop myself and try again. I have not accepted defeat in this matter as yet. In time, I hope they will join me, as it took time to make them realize their worth and to not give up.

I feel isolated very often, and this is increasing with time but I cannot find any solution. I don't want to watch porn, cheesy videos or YouTube to beat the feeling. Instead, I want company and some responsibility, to feel worthy again for a change.

Whenever (and it is very, very rare) I meet my friends, I start with the topic of TBI which only I can relate to. That probably distances me from them. They may expect me to talk about other, more interesting stuffs, but this is my reality (partially). And I believe that with friends and family we are expected to talk our heart out and express our true feelings.

The time gap between my injury, until now has created a gap in many areas: education, independence, and having responsibility. There is a gap of maturity and self-realization which is really hard to understand and discuss.

There's no way out except rigorous workouts and therapy but, years later you find yourself trapped. Sometimes other work helps you flourish and rejuvenate. It boosts your stamina and capacity, pushing you and taking to you to a different level. I feel squeezed, frustrated and trapped again in my schedule. It is like it is closing in on my opportunities to grow. I keep reminding myself of never giving up but I'm bored of repetition and angered by not getting it right.

All left within is anger: the anger of failure not seen by others, the feeling of helplessness at not being understood and perceived wrongly. Feeling handicapped feels I have lost an integral part of me all these years. Like some limbs are uncoordinated, there's no stability in the behaviour as well. My mood sways much more than anyone can think of. Self-maligning and cursing myself is my biggest drawback as well as an advantage. Occasionally, it encourages me to grab more out of me.

I am assailable from every angle, and to change this I must bring a major change within. I must give up on anger, frustration and cribbing. I am not a winner but a loser who finds shelter in 'shouting'. My weaknesses are plenty; my strength, none. I cannot handle the depression and frustration that arise out of my daily routine and I'm really tired of the scars of past protruding out from every effort I make. I am trying and willing myself to be happy but it seems like an impossible and farfetched task.

Occasionally, I meet people who make me feel ecstatic and ignite certain hope, but it is later extinguished.

***

Everyone needs someone, perhaps for discussion or sometimes, just to talk and release the negative enzymes that are present in abundance inside the body.

My family understand me very well because they know where I have arisen from, and they see potential in me. Also, they have suffered along with me. It's not only the person who suffers a dreadful injury who undergoes all the difficulties I have been writing about; the family of the survivor experiences the same.

Brain injury brings you closer to your family. No one else actually has the time to listen and pay attention to your thoughts and emotions, but family always stay around. Friends are there but for a short while. As time passes by they all get busy; you cannot blame them as they also have a life to live. I always tell myself, 'it's my journey and I have to travel it alone'. It's like a self-motivating quote.

All love has an expiry date – except mother love. It's not that mother keeps you hidden from reality but she is able to put things in a comforting way. She has to balance her love between all family members as they are all equal from her point of view, and sometimes a harshness in her voice might hurt you, but she is only trying to balance her selfless love. No one can actually understand your pain, shallowness, inferiority and depression but my mother's aim is to make me, the survivor and victim, realize the importance of keeping on trying and following the prescribed path for betterment. (Even she sometimes fails to realise the misery of my life however, because dependency sometimes extends too far.)

I have learned to find peace, tolerance and companionship in myself. With others, including family, I was being judged and given directions. If I refused to do what they said, I turned into the bad guy, whereas on my own I could make mistakes and rectify them. I have also realized that my protective shield is not needed every time, although there is a constant fear of getting hurt, even by your parents.

Family-get-togethers are harder. I know my family well, even extended family and relations, but people tend to forget what I'm capable of and ask me stupid questions like, "Do you recognize me?" and, "What is my name?" When I go to family functions, I try my best to look and act normal but my walk and speech defy me. I feel more self-conscious, and there are more gaffes. I recently realized when you're over-prepared you tend to make more mistakes and feel degraded.

Over the years not many of my relatives came to visit me during my difficult time of struggle. I meet them only at family functions. It would be good if they behaved cordially, but sometimes their questions make me feel distant from them. I'm actually distant from many.

Looking at the brighter side of this, I have come closer to my immediate family, sharing my thoughts with them about things which I never discussed or even mentioned before. I am now more attached to my family than before, talking with them, going out with them, and saying what I feel and think.

The **topic of expenses** is a raw one. My parents and family spent so much money on getting me home, and helping me recover. When I think about the amounts, I feel squinched. I almost feel I owe them two lives. They avoid the question of 'how much', answering it buoyantly, making us all glow. However, as a survivor, I am very much aware of where and how much I spend.

***

Caregivers are the real survivors. They behave and act normally in front of the sufferers, but they sacrifice a part of their life every time they are dealing with a person with brain injury. We, the sufferers rather than survivors, often fail to understand their condition and mental state. They are usually on the receiving end of all the drama, anger, pain and helplessness of the sufferer.

Who are these 'givers' of 'care'? We are not always familiar with the term 'caregiver'. Essentially, caregivers are people who sacrifice everything for the sufferer who has been affected by trauma. They are the real survivors because they live their life in accordance with someone else's needs, limiting their own personal growth for the sake of the person who is actually born again.

The sufferer, experiencing everything around him or her changing, is often unaware of the circumstances of the caregivers. We are unaware that they are sacrificing their social circles and the limelight they used to experience before, boycotting themselves from the outside world.

Caregivers have their own emotions but they never show them because of the sufferer. They know their tears, worries or fears will affect the sufferer. No doctor or therapist can understand the suffering and the feelings of the sufferer better than the caregivers. They see the growth of the sufferer at every level. They feel the emotions behind the sufferer's anger, frustrations and smiles. They see the tears which they hide behind their jolly faces, which actually come from fear of losing everyone around them, their loved ones.

The victims are so busy fighting their own battles, that they cannot feel the emotions of the caregivers who are putting their own lives at stake. Everyone is so busy counselling the sufferer that they often neglect the real survivors, the caregivers.

***

Something I have learned from my life after TBI is this: as humans, we are most affected by the word 'they'. Sometimes we are inspired by 'them', the big names we often see on television or read in the newspaper. We do not envy them but it inspires and motivates us in some way or the other. More often, though, 'they' have a negative effect on us.

Who are 'they'? They are the people we always see around us. In fact, we are surrounded by them. 'They' affect us both consciously and unconsciously, and often our future plans are decided and executed after thinking, "What will 'they' say?"

Will 'they' make fun of us or appreciate us?

If 'they' can do it, why can't we?

We postpone or cancel plans after thinking would 'they' have done the same or not? What would 'they' say? How would 'they' interpret something? We get nervous thinking over and over in our head about 'them'.

Our world revolves around 'them', not our loved ones but others. The consequences that follow from that are that sometimes we do not follow our mind or our heart. Instead, we follow fear.

But 'they' will never understand us and the emptiness inside us which is not visible in this competitive world, with those competitive glares present everywhere. They feel they know us and understand us but they don't. They see our faces and think we are lonely but we are not, we all actually have many friends but not a single one with whom we can share our thoughts or someone who understands us.

'They' make us feel inferior as 'they' see us as a person who needs help in everything. They never realise that they are making us hate them and giving us a bad impression of themselves. They don't become superior humans in our eyes by 'helping', and we still hate them for interfering unnecessarily or helping without our consent.

I feel that caring for someone makes the person on the receiving end feel good, but deciding for that person disgusts them. It instils a feeling of exclusion. Consoling someone afterwards is hypocrisy.

We are always looking for friendship with the cool guys but 'cool' people are the most uncool ones in real life. After my accident I have faced some very bitter realities. It is as if I am face to face with the reality of life, where I see the true colours of everyone – and they are not always beautiful. The time I invested in cool and unworthy people, I now wish I had invested in more meaningful activities and people. I would surely be in a lot better position and state of mind.

I struggle in not being appreciated by others. I sweat, but not due to scarcity of water. I burn not to be titled as the next ghost-rider. I mumble not because I am scared or hungry. I avoid meeting people because I know their reactions might displease me and my actions might go wrong and distance them.

I am not a bunch of mistakes who is dying for acceptance: I ask for regular behaviour and nothing extra. I'm well aware of my limitations and I very well know where I lack. It is like living in a reality show where everyone sympathises you and continues to do so.

I have seen sympathizing faces; trust me, I don't need them. All I need is cordial behaviour and no help where it is not required. The result of all this sympathy has made me to avoid asking for help, even at places where it is required.

I am working, not to be accepted by others the way I am, but because I have a hope of walking with them. I'm not hoping for praise, just the normality I used to get. I feel insulted and shallow in the company of others as well as myself. I cannot take pride in what I have overcome and overpowered because whenever I step outside I am scared of insult and embarrassment, which I may invite despite being continually very cautious and aware of my actions and surroundings.

The positive points might be few but thankfully, they are present. Realizing who is with you and for you in this long race, supporting you throughout, shatters the mask they have been wearing. When you go deeper with them, you feel you actually never knew this person before.

There are people who want to help; they should help the needy who ask for help. Others want to help, but they will only help those who are well-dressed and, if they speak, speak decently or in a proper fluency.

India is an emerging nation and hopefully will emerge as one of the most powerful nations but we all need to value other individuals. Everyone carries a certain honour and self-respect in themselves. We have no right to hurt it. I have done it several times but today I feel very ashamed and guilty of it. Primarily, we need to emerge and grow as individuals and look beyond financial and physical appearance.

Chapter Six

On My Own

I have been dragging myself along from the very first day since little I knew and understood about the Traumatic Brain Injury. I have worked day and night to reach a point where I can walk alone, go out and live life independently, albeit still needing some support.

It would be really easy to blame my friends for my loneliness but I have to understand their situation. They are in a similar situation to me; the difference is that I am struggling to live a life that looks 'normal', while they are struggling to make a future. When we face the truth that nothing lasts forever, it is a reality check. I am going through a different phase in my life, in which I am experiencing all the feelings at once, without intervals.

When we were living back in the twentieth century, with the excitement of entering the twenty-first century with its advanced communication and technology, we never realized that we would get so busy and mean, and would distance ourselves from one another.

No one likes being alone but with my health deficiency I am forced to be alone. With time, everything starts falling apart and I experience living in a world you could never imagine.

I have reached a point where I have no one to share my feelings with. It may just be that I have a lack of confidence, or perhaps, that I am being immature and this is a feeling speaking, not my conscious and sound mind. My mind swirls with the possibilities and I feel like I am being taken over by loneliness and even going mad.

***

I love Mondays! Perhaps I'm unlike most people, but I like weekdays because on those days I have a planned schedule. I stay motivated and involved in my therapy and exercises, and have the option to go to the office. I am not bored as I am involved in something. I just have to keep control over certain things, and keep myself under my command if I wish to make each day worth living.

However, it's up and down. Some weekdays are good: I have good speech (some days), and I feel confident in myself, but some are awfully bad, with bad speech and self-doubt.

I hate weekends. They add to my feelings of being useless, alone and helpless. I cannot help myself much, and my relationships with my friends have been on halt for years. All holidays, in fact, are difficult because I have no companionship and being on my own is quite depressing, giving rise to unwanted thoughts. I get bored, feeling futile and ineffective. Sundays draw out the worst in me, fighting with my parents (as I have control only over them), but it damages my relationship with them reputation, and I curse myself later.

I think a lot, mainly on weekends or whenever I have no work. In my mind, I'm busy defending myself, proving I can do things. 'Let me try,' I say to people in my head. At times, I feel as if I'm confined to my own thoughts, hurling abuse, but even then, a silent, high-pitched voice within says, "No matter what, just don't give up."

We must help one another, and for once, make someone feel secure, not guiding them until asked, and not imposing on them our ideas. Everyone has someone to teach but we may not understand their problems until we are in their shoes, so think before you speak and give suggestions.

Chapter Seven

Self worth

Sometimes I feel like an over grown toddler, following my parents through shopping malls or grocery stores. I want to purchase something but I hold myself back, because I have a question in my head: 'Am I really worth it?'

Self-worth may be understood in innumerable ways. You're 'worthy' because you contribute to society. You're not worthy because you are expensive to keep. Maybe you don't deserve that item. Maybe you could buy it yourself, but you can't have it if your parents are paying. Should I just be content with myself? The thoughts go around and around, and my many questions pester me, making it difficult to breathe and think, and remaining unanswered.

When people treat me as if I am not a part of their world, it affects the way I see myself. I don't need extra care and help from them; all I need is acceptance, the way I am. I get cheerful meeting known people, disheartened when people meet me, but after seeing me walking and talking, they change their attitude towards me and suddenly become more cautious. They start 'helping' me and do not even try to understand me. Instead, they ask the person next to me to repeat what I've said, which is very annoying and disappointing at the same time. When I do meet people who treat me normally, and not like a patient, it's hard to appreciate it, because my mind is still stuck in previous situations and comparison begins.

Traumatic Brain Injury perhaps isn't the sole reason that I face social difficulties/ awkwardness. Attention Deficit Disorder, which was a feature of my earlier life, is a serious disorder, with the consequence that you start living to impress complete strangers. (Hyperactivity is neutral – it brings certain advantages and disadvantages, some of which are feeling incompetent within.)

Sometimes – in fact, many times – I feel like crying; I'm being left behind in the human race of actually growing up and being independent. It feels shameful to discuss this with anyone as everyone thinks I am not the type of person who would crib over such petty issues.

I write things down, to help my thoughts, but it's always on this topic. My family asks me to write about something else but how can I, when this is the only thing in my mind, always wondering how life would have been if my accident had not happened, and how can anyone accept this?

Guilt is an underrated feeling in terms of its effect. Guilt ruins a person from the inside. Guilt runs throughout the body, despite the fact that we keep assuring ourselves that we *aren't* guilty, and we keep denying the feeling. I am guilty of incidents that had happened in the past – things that tore me apart and brought me here. I am guilty of going against the wishes of my loved ones. I carry the guilt of not being able to adjust in my shoes in which I have travelled earlier, travelled long. I am guilty of not being able to look beyond the limitations that my fear and mind have conceived. I am guilty of not being as good as everyone expects me to be, of not performing as well as friends and family expect.

I don't want to be the mentor whom everyone looks up to. With so many people watching me, waiting for results, I feel imprisoned, and cannot think freely. People say they do not care about how well I do, but I know results matter. Indeed, I grew up in an environment where results matter more than anything; results change how people look at you.

I don't know where I am lacking, but, it's obvious that I lack, as people don't accept me, for reasons which are invisible to me. They still behave like they are dealing with someone who does not belong amongst them. When two persons are conversing, they look towards each other and pay attention to the other; this doesn't happen when people converse with me. I often feel I am miles away from being normal and this behaviour is going to defeat me, and make me fall but I feel within myself, that if I fall this time, it would be really tough to get up and gather all the pieces. Maybe I just need to be treated like my old version ~~of~~ was treated ~~before~~, and then I'll rise and will be more comfortable. But I like new version of me.

In normal life, we get a sense of worth from work, but when you have no work or responsibility, it makes no difference whether you stay at home or go to the office. When people from your own family cannot give you attention and make you realize your importance, you cannot expect the outside world to accept you and treat you any differently.

Now, after spending much time feeling useless and like I'm a waste item that is practically of no use, I wonder, 'Why did God save me? Was it to show me my real worth?' Well, at present, it does not exist. In that case, my accident was surely a lesson, which clearly meant 'Respect what I gave you.'

I should be happy that I have been given an opportunity to live again but I regret it most of the time, because I don't deserve the negative treatment I get. I cannot live with it and will never accept it.

In simple words, I sum it up by saying, 'Shit happened and it is happening again, over time.'(the behaviour)

The thought of committing suicide has crossed my mind at various points, but I have stopped myself. 'You are not a coward who would surrender,' I tell myself, and I think of my family, who are happy seeing me breathing every day, and trying to live.

I visited a noble man who said that you shall not search for happiness. Instead be happy and joyful from the inside and happiness shall come to you. Is that really applicable in the real world? Are you supposed to just hear what people say and ignore it? I have not yet attained such peace where I'm able to hear, ignore and not mind later.

I tend to find comfort in grief as I am discovering new things and new capabilities about myself every passing day. I take pride in over-coming challenges and embrace them with a grin.

Chapter Eight

Fate and life

I never blame destiny for what has happened. I can either live in my past and feel disgusted about it or work to make my future flawless and bright. However, I do wish I would have thought of the consequences before I sat on the parapet. Perhaps none of this would have ever happened.

The consequences have been significant. I often feel embarrassed at the way I speak and feel very small when I am not able to explain myself, even in a situation which I know and understand very well. I am losing my confidence because I fail in everything I do, explaining things to others. I am way too conscious about everything and all this is because of my speech and my posture. I look broken and I am scared of taking responsibility, or managing things.

When it seems like life has come to a dead end, and you cannot see any way out, you are trapped. You cannot escape, and it feels like your thoughts are killing you. This is truly what brain injury is all about, fighting with your own self, and realizing the value of life and its importance.

Years after my Traumatic Brain Injury, I have truly realized the value of life. It is not about getting a job, getting a degree to show off or establishing a business. Life is about being fit and healthy and independent. Please God, give me and all of us the power to stay strong, happy, loving and caring.

I and my family have been through the worst but this doesn't make much of a difference. Everyone is dealing with their own struggles in life. Perhaps their struggles might look easier than mine from outside, but that may just be because of their invisible and unnoticed persistence.

I keep thinking that I am suffering the most but it is not true. My family has been through a lot, but they still smile and encourage me. They have put restrictions on their normal lives for my benefit and make sacrifices for my good, but their efforts often go unnoticed and neglected because I still take out all my frustrations and anger on them. Sometimes I feel like a volcano, releasing all its heat and lava on others without being affected by myself.

I am in no way a particularly moral soul but I have come to realise some important things because of my situation. We live in a world where a person's worth is determined by seeing positives and pointing out the negatives. But pointing out the negatives is like scratching a wound; it doesn't help in healing it. Instead, it makes it more severe by undermining and discouraging the healing process.

I have realised the importance of family, who are often taken for granted. My trusted friends walked away from me, busy in their respective lives, or using the term 'busy' as an excuse to shed the burden.

I have realised the importance of God-given ability, perception and mobility. Mine are not as quick as they were, but I have realised that where there's a will there's definitely a way.

I have realised the importance of learning; it helps in every stage of life, lifting you up and giving you assurance. Unfortunately one of the saddest parts of my brain injury is that I often forget things. Retention is one of my hardest tasks. When I keep looking for words or sentences again and again, it makes me feeble.

I have realised that only we are responsible for our own happiness. It is the only way to enlightenment; the joy and peace we find within prospers us.

I often see posts on the TBI support group that say something like, 'You cannot understand the sufferings, feelings and pain we endure until you go through the same'. I have repeated this myself, out of frustration, but when I think deeply, I realize that this is not what I want others to experience. Rather, I would prefer to spread awareness about Traumatic Brain Injury. I want to break the absurd silence which I and others experience towards our situation.

Spreading awareness about TBI can only be done by talking about it. It does no good to keep feeling ashamed and hating oneself. In spreading awareness, I hope to get to know more people with brain injury and develop a support system which is more useful and favourable than constantly being surrounded by people who judge and comment without any knowledge.

No one knows about anything until they or their loved ones experience the suffering but, the aim here is to make more and more people know about TBI, and connect care givers and survivors. It feels so good walking down the stairs, taking the escalators, being the newer improved version of the new you, doing things which were earlier heavier tasks. Appreciation and overcoming things is much more than a pat on back.

TBI has given me courage, wisdom, patience, tolerance, and acceptance. Patience is a part of accepting the harsh truth and reality of life, with peace to fulfil your desires. TBI has helped me learn the 'weird stare', intimidating spectators before they apply same trick on me.

With time and experience, and having faced the scariest nightmare and put in continuous efforts for a better tomorrow, I sometimes think I have forgotten to live in the present. The present is where we belong as humans – neither in the past, nor the future. Sometimes, however, events that happened in the past leave you doomed in the present, wondering what to do or wondering what's happening around you.

It's as if you're just walking without directions or a map. And if you appear different from what people around you perceive of you, you will be on the receiving side forever, till you establish yourself into something bigger and better.

It's not being lonely or mostly ignored, that is the cause of my disbelief in myself. The cause of this is how strangers perceive me. I feel embarrassed and out of place no matter where I go. Everyone is undermining me, making me feel enervated and debilitated.

Chapter Nine

Depression

Post TBI, I have suffered from insomnia and sleepless nights because of the guilt of losing myself. I think deeply on mistakes I've made in the past; they are embarrassing and cannot be corrected and redone. I feel concerned about things that are out of my control and situations that are unacceptable, about which people have no reaction or comments other than showing sympathy. Sometimes, or even most of the time, things seem in hand and can be managed but then it's easier to let them slip, which creates a mess and changes plans and goals.

The day we are born, we begin planning. By the time we become independent, we indulge in making plans for ourselves, but we rarely think of consequences of actions which might reverse everything, bring us back to being dependent and make us feel lonely. We never imagine that we might will once again be a person who requires assistance often but fears or avoid asking for it.

We exist, not just to breathe and eat, but, to make a reputation and earn a living. When we can't do that, life seems aimless and purposeless. Life is like tap without water. We sing songs we like (unless we are in an orchestra or performing for money). We do activities that make us happy, bringing out the positives in us which propel us to do well.

I feel sick watching kids of my age cursing life and focusing on negativity instead of appreciating the fact that they are alive, experiencing appreciating the good. Good things in life might be limited but they exist, and will multiply if you neglect all the negative thoughts. Think good and good will come.

Adapting or accepting? These words might look like synonyms, and it can be tough differentiating between the two, as both are a different part of the same answer, but let's see how they might differ.

When someone adapts to situation they work towards improvement, betterment of themselves and procuring good. In contrast, when they accept a situation, they are bound by restrictions. They carry on, cursing their destiny and leave the healing to time, forgetting that time heals only when we work and utilize it.

'Accepting' a situation is equivalent to kneeling down to circumstances. You are 'accepting' the new you – the weak you, the dependent you and the vulnerable you. Adapting to a situation gives you another opportunity to accept things and mould them so that they are better. Accepting is laying down your weapons and surrendering, while adapting is fighting from within and trying to defeat your barriers in life.

Depression, grief and agony are things I must fight all the time. Depression comes from the suffering of conveying my message in a way that makes me look helpless and degraded. Grief gives rise to debilitating thoughts, and agony ends all feelings. It makes me sceptical about everything that exists, and I think that there is nothing interesting or effective happening in life.

There's a kind of insecurity in my voice. I'm often terrified, giving a lot of thought before finally speaking, and later I find myself explaining as to why I said something. I think I'm quite unsure of my status and position. It's not only my voice, but my actions and reactions that depict an uncertain me. I am like a curious, inquisitive and impatient teenager who still cribs (to himself though) for attention, importance and anger. However, I avoid company and seclude myself as others see me as a responsibility, who needs to be taken care of, generating sympathy or compassion which I cannot stand. I am trying hard to impress people instead of living, but this actually pushes me down the drain leaving me undecided and gloomy. At the beginning of last year, my resolution was to inculcate myself with positivity from within. Negativity is a curse, eating you from inside out, and reminding you only of all your impediments.

I decided to focus on accomplishable and feasible goals in the months that would follow, and accompany them with patience, discipline and positivity. I pledged to breathe in positivity and to pump my heart and brain with positive vibes. I do not wish to limit my happiness because of the impediments in my way, or the judgement of others, who make efforts to swipe you off your feet and don't pay attention towards you. You gotta stand tough! I am not scared of dying but living has become a challenge for me.

In the entire journey through the years, I realised I am not sad, just unhappy. It took longer than usual to realise the discrepancy in my behaviour, which is good to an extent but afterwards leads to defamation and self-maligning. A man can have everything he desires but he must adapt to new challenge and changes; change is both appreciable and frustrating. Change filters body with positive as well as negative elements, which both restrict you to a certain level. Who you've become can be the opposite of what you were, which invites both applause and criticism. You are happy and unhappy sometimes and confused often.

Despite the happiness you are trying to infuse in you, the monotonous relationship you have entered into with your restricted life is frustrating. You never want to remind yourself of limitations but they keep coming back, especially on weekends and holidays. This is the time when you lose your already weak calm and composure self.

I feel like a dormant volcano which is quiet because of weakness, but which wants to explode with the answers that my conscious mind utters silently. I feel okay, but not expressive enough. I want to break the shackles and erase the debilitating thoughts which make me a sissy who is weak from within.

I start my day happy but as the hours progress I enter into conversation with people from different walks of life and their perception of myself fills me with negativity and depression. Sometimes the negativity helps me to speak at a slow pace and realise the benefits of what has happened in the last few hours or minutes. The positive side of negativity is that it allows me to adapt to the reality of how things are meant to be done. During this small phase, as soon as things start going in my favour, I become exhilarated and ruin it all again which makes me negative. The drawbacks of negativity are destroying my relationship with people, and making me mumble about 'how should have I said that?' All in all negativity is neither beneficial nor helpful except in teaching me to speak slowly.

Whenever I'm sad I pledge to look at the brighter side. I miss my old self when I look back on my memories, and make some unrealistic commitments to myself. Not finding yourself perfect for any work because there might be certain restrictions on you that leave you baffled. You are constantly straining to be happy, to love yourself, and to embrace the present but you feel incomplete in almost every situation. I experience mood swings more than any one you can think of, and the bad days are so bad that they make me feel worse than criminals guilty of abduction and rape.

Chapter Ten

My Future

If I say I am not thinking much about my future it wouldn't be true. This accident changed my plans, but not my goals in life, and I have become very stubborn. My goal was to become a self-made person, an achiever in life and it is still the same. If one option closes, plenty of others open.

I am a very opportunistic person and I believe that God must have thought of something better for me in life, if he has put this incident in the books for me. I want to concentrate on getting back in shape and to be independent. I want to drive my car, walk my dog and do plenty of other stuffs. I don't want to be dependent on others for anything.

At the age of 21 many young people start earning or running their own businesses. At the age of 21, I was learning how to balance and how to talk. But my day will come, I have faith in God and myself.

However, I am very confused and concerned regarding my future because I don't know what I will do. Before my accident, I was pursuing a five year Law program. I was forced to quit it after five semesters because of my accident. I have begun going back, but now I am losing interest in law.

Being a TBI survivor, I am not proud of myself that I am working so hard, as anyone would do the same. I am just worried about my future. But I keep telling myself, "Nothing is in your hands. It's God who decides everything. All we humans can do is just dream and make plans. It's he who does the execution."

Post Traumatic Brain Injury, my personal interests have not changed but they have been delayed as I face my various challenges. My focus has certainly shifted to recovery. In terms of achieving and earning I feel stuck. My brain has created a paradox beyond which I cannot think. I want to reach far but I do not want to put the blame on the irregularities in me. I have options in mind but they close on me as I see myself incomplete. My main goal is reaching out to people, creating awareness and making them understand the situation I am in.

When I see updates on social networking sites about people I know getting jobs and hanging out, I feel left out. After a while, I am back to my normal self but the feeling is not gone. It has sunk inside somewhere, buried deep down. However, I don't let it affect me negatively and I try to push myself and achieve all that is left behind. Time that has passed cannot be brought back but a new script can be written every passing day.

I do not know what interests me, but I want to do something which is engrossing. Sitting at home and doing nothing is a failure in itself. I have never been the kind of person who sits home all day long, and does nothing. It eats me up inside.

Writing has been very helpful to me. Jotting down my feelings is good but it's hard to stay positive. My writing pattern depends on how my day has been. The misery-stricken parts of me jerk out and make my writing sound like I'm begging for sympathy. Also, I find that all my writing seems to revolve around the injury, but I am the epicentre here, not my injury.

It's hard to think about the idea of me publishing a book and people reading it. I don't want sympathy from anyone, especially if they feel they might have wronged me or hurt me. It's for both of us to realise our respective faults and not to try to re-do things. Just let it be.

I accompany my father to his office often, but there I see myself as an adult kid who is curious about everything but scared to ask questions because everyone might get a wrong interpretation and perception. My speech also plays a negative role here but I feel good and occupied for some time. Even doing just a little amount of work gives me happiness. I didn't realise that even just six months of going with my father would give me such happiness. A little bit of work uplifts my confidence in self, and when this happens, I am busy browsing web searching fruitful courses. I think of letting go and letting things settle on their own but I'm quite certain of my age and the fear of failure. I'm not disheartened but scared of having nothing in my hands. I wish to seize the day but insecurities about the future keep my mind busy and insecure.

Joining college again was definitely a good decision, but when returning to college, I had a different perspective. I remembered my old college days, convivial, and filled with fun, but I was not able to adjust to the new environment because of certain limitations in me. I made new friends, all five years younger than me, and within a day and after much interaction, I realized that college kids these days were much more practical than we ever were. After a few days, meeting a few more people I concluded that people like me used to (funny, extrovert) exist, but in a much lower ratio than before. It was difficult to find anyone who made me feel at home.

After a while, I began to see that the college kids, while quite practical in the way they talked, were very immature in the way they thought. Yes, they were kind and helpful in behaviour, but I found that if you were not as fast, talkative and quick witted as them, they would distance you, or move away. Sometimes there were exceptions and you will also find people who will use you or your weakness and you will never realise it. I don't mean to say they are bad, but very smart – much smarter than you were. They know a side of life which many are unable to see, or they see it but never act on it.

Not all people born in the later generation are clever and practical but the majority is. In earlier years, kids would make fun of people who were different, and would never understand the limitations that one faces. The present generation, however, understands and letting go is not that difficult for them.

Am I enjoying college? I cannot find a good reason to explain why, but I am not. It has just become an escape from my daily routine and to avoid questions about my speech and balance and 'what happened to him?'

Do qualifications matter? Let's find out by listening in on a conversation between two strangers probably living in the same community, but meeting for the first time:

A: Hi.

B: Hi, how are you?

A: I am good, thank you. How are you?

B: I am good too, thank you. What do you do for a living? What are your qualifications?

A: I am recovering/haven't found suitable profession yet/confused about what I really like/have some limitations. I passed school in 2008, thereafter was pursuing law but met with an accident in 2011 and was on a sabbatical for four years. I have been busy with my recovery, doing therapy to get back in shape. I started back at my old college this year; they were generous to take me back but since I have started I am not enjoying it. My class mates are quite understanding, but it's difficult to gel with them because of my limitation and speech issues. I think they are quite nice but at the end of the day it's all about personal capabilities.

I have my exams from Monday but I haven't prepared much as I keep on forgetting. Actually, I am not that interested this time. But, sorry I kept speaking and forgot about you.

B: I think you have done pretty good with your recovery and you look fine. A little more work required on speech and you will be as good as new. I think you must continue your law and finish it, as being a graduate is important. I have to go. I will catch you later. Byee, and take care. God bless you.

A (to himself): I think it's all about how you look from the outside. Your personal views will only be entertained if you look good and presentable. I wish I could do something for the people suffering like me or experiencing the same phase in their life.

This is how long a conversation lasts between a qualified person and not-so-qualified person. There are already several barriers that keep people at a distance from one another. I hope this scenario doesn't emerge as another barrier.

As a kid I never thought at all about what it means to be a graduate. Do we value people for who they are as individuals or for what they emerge as, including their qualification, income and social status? I have several troubles. I am not trying to be a hero by highlighting them and discussing them openly, but will it make any difference if I sit at home, hiding, and being afraid of talking about it?

Part of my increasing independence has been to get back on board of the Metro service in my city. Getting on board again was something I always wanted to do. Asking others to drop me places, or taking private cabs was not feasible and made me feel enfeebled and handicapped. Plus, the Metro helped me to get out of my comfort zone and gain some confidence. I wanted to break the zone of dependency my mind had created.

I started back on the Metro after I had gained the complete confidence in myself, knew my strengths and weaknesses and was ready to handle hurdles. I didn't face many jaw-clenching moments except at connecting stations which are usual on my route. The Metro is constructed beautifully and if you reach it early, it gives you the time to work out and burn some fat as you to have walk a lot. (Although there are elevators and escalators.)

Travelling on the Metro has been good for me. The strangers there don't stare with doubtful, questioning, or pitying faces. Metro very rarely gives you a chance to relax because there's too much crowd; one barely gets the chance to stand alone even in the elevator. It gives you the opportunity to run into people whom you haven't seen in years. It also gives you exposure to new routes, different stations and the latest schemes the DMRC is running. Travelling in Metro alone also boosts your confidence, encourages you and increases self-belief. There are minor struggles with my speech but inside the Metro one rarely speaks. In contrast, interacting with auto/rickshaw vendors is equivalent to talking to an adolescent with little or no knowledge and, mind you, they aren't cute.

My future is full of predictability and probability. It's good that I live such a predictable life because everything is planned and pre-decided. But it's boring too, as nothing's entertaining. Daily, I face the same mourning over my speech, never feeling content with whatever little I have achieved, never feeling proud of breaking the shackles, and feeling restricted every time I decide to do something. I feel paranoid whenever I want to take a step further and not confident regarding anything whatsoever.

All of this just because I'm ashamed whenever I'm intending to speak. I know many can't speak. But I'm joyous for that small achievement. I'm not trying to belittle myself but my expectations are high, knowing I have come a good distance from where I was. I have read and heard that progress post-TBI is slow, but I don't wish to be slow! I'm exhausted by reading inspiring, motivational and uplifting stories as I trust only mine. Those stories are true and very real but I wish to make my own, and then believe in reality and destiny. It has been years and I very well know the reactions of people as to how they'll behave and react, both near ones and outsiders. Still, though, I react to their reactions, frequently and almost daily. I need to inculcate calmness, politeness and patience in myself to obstruct such reactions and be formidable in my reception of others. Self-belief and confidence in an individual is an investment in oneself. If the same amount of belief and confidence that he puts in himself is shown by his peers he will work harder to prosper.

The probability of getting good treatment post-trauma is not predictable because there are only a certain number of trauma centres and therapists. Just having a degree doesn't make an efficient therapist; to find one possessing both qualification and talent is a blessing which is equivalent to spotting a meteorite.

Whether or not you will be self-dependant is neither predictable nor probable, but totally dependent on how one maintains their composure. Thinking negative is predictable; the probability of thinking positive is a hard task to achieve.

The probability of people praising and motivating you is high: the same people predicting about what you shall do now is also high.

About me, a prediction might say, "It has been so many years and there won't be any further improvement." But I'm probable of making certain changes in myself by adapting to changes which are necessary for a better outcome. So for me recovery is ongoing.

When one is suffering from a chronic injury or Traumatic Brain Injury, how you were or how you are at present isn't important. All that counts is how far you have come and your potential to keep on going. You might encounter many defeats but you must not be defeated.

I am not stuck in the past. But the vulnerability I carry forward from my past into the present worries me. I've composed and moulded myself to be able to live in the present, regardless of the pressures on me. I am thankful to my past for giving me another try and thankful to the present for accepting me.

Do I blame the past or the present for my difficulties? The past was my 'present' on that severe day of my accident – the day that broke me. This helps me to grasp that it wasn't the past or the present that is to blame. What happened came about because of a bad decision. Knowing this has given me the will to take control rather than blaming the past or the present. Taking a silly risk was my choice and working on it today is my choice as well. Of course, though, it's hard that in the meantime I get panic attacks that freak me out and make me lose determination.

Transferring blame is an easier job but taking the blame on my own is maturity. It is now that I have realised the foolishness and immaturity of the act that landed me in an abyss. TBI has taught me maturity. I have realised it's not worth answering every query that people make of me, and especially about 'what happened', because people are too curious to find out what's going on in others' lives rather than enjoying their own. I keep my issues to myself because there's a great saying: "You know yourself the best."

Chapter Eleven

Happiness

Both happiness and sadness are a part and package of the journey we all know as 'life'. The former involves effort while the latter follows at various stages of life.

I have realized and accepted that there's no fun in participation if you aren't joyous within. First and foremost, we have to attain peace with ourselves and embrace life, without expectation from anyone other than ourselves. Let us impregnate ourselves with happiness, feel content with what we currently hold and strive for more for a regular flow.

Life is a short journey; be enthralled with happiness and do not make it shallow with grief. Sometimes, we are a puzzle that is scattered into pieces. Reassembling the pieces drives you crazy; happiness might help to keep them within reach and accessible.

Happiness is your key to anything and everything you desire. It won't make your journey easy but it will definitely be smoother. I know it is a tough task to feel jubilant always. It is a practice which one has to infuse with learning to let go. A time will come when you are alone but do not let it make you helpless, dependent on circumstances and others for your happiness. You are strong, and capable of facing and enduring challenges! You were given this life and will succeed, not immediately but eventually.

Worrying is a waste of time. It doesn't change anything. It messes with your mind and steals your happiness. Be like the great Sachin Tendulkar: let your actions do the talking.

It is easy to smile with a camera pointed at you but we are not happy unless we get a good picture. The introduction of front facing cameras with which we could take 'selfies', put the control in our hands. Similarly, our key to happiness lies with us and within us. We can expect more of ourselves, but we cannot rely on anyone else, no matter who they are.

It is other people's views about you that hamper your happiness most, whether those people are known or unknown to you. People unknown to you know nothing about your struggle, situation and circumstances and yet still have questions and suggestions for you. Those who know you often fail to understand you; they have no idea of the storm you are experiencing and you fail the expectations they may have of you. I am sure you expect more from yourself than anyone else does.

We all try to follow our hearts for our own happiness but we still think a lot about others' happiness and peace. My conclusion? Redeem your happiness from the burden of anyone else's expectations – anyone other than yourself. Beauty is about living your life, being happy with yourself inside out and not worrying about what people think of you.

Your thoughts stay and travel with you. If they are focused on damaging your reputation, disturbing your peace and being self-maligning, they stay for a longer period. Try accommodating them so that they lift you higher, boost you, motivate you and inspire you rather than stealing your happiness and peace.

You might feel helpless in certain situations and assume negativity is driving the person you are dealing with. At these times, being happy and positive sounds unachievable, but carrying them along in your backpack helps in unpacking. Happiness lies in not accepting the defeat, nor succumbing to the circumstances nor resisting to the fear of failure.

It has been a long time since I enjoyed a careless sleep. My brain is always provoking me to try harder, knowing there's nothing more I can do except to incorporate happiness and never give up in life. Satisfaction with your current effort and regime adds to happiness.

I do not wish to be known or remembered by the very few people who know me as 'an ordinary guy who tried but did not go the extra mile'. I want them to remember me as 'the guy who sustained serious injuries, who never gave up but still couldn't make it'. I don't want to be the guy who kept thinking of accomplishing a lot but never had the courage or willingness to go the extra mile which could win me accolades.

I do not wish to spend nights cursing myself for something I did not try, because I did not have the courage or just because of my laid-back nature and sense of self-inferiority. I want to erase all this reluctance in this, my second chance at life and hope to come up with good. Yes, it is a tedious journey but it gives me enthusiasm and pleasure to overcome challenges and tough tasks. At this age, I am often saddened with the agony of not being able to reach milestones in life. I want to be happy but something keeps me occupied with grief even when my mind is inviting happiness and joy. I often fail to understand the journey which has become a part of my life. Here I must train my brain to abstain from paying attention to words, phrases or statements that degrade my existence, journey and struggle.

This is the hardest thing I have come across, post-Traumatic Brain Injury, because healing a heart is much more difficult than healing a damaged brain. I am never tired in my exercise periods. But being happy and joyous within is genuinely hard. I want to cry and get rid of all the toxins within so that I can smile without the regret of guilt in me. The strongest feeling of guilt comes from not enjoying life, making some bad choices and not making my parents proud of me.

We all were born individuals (even those of us who are twins) but later became trapped by the burden of making a living and a future for us, our family and our spouse. Somewhere along the line we neglected happiness, with the burden of bettering our standard of living and lifestyle. I'm not saying you should neglect your choices of having a healthy lifestyle, just, along with that, be happy.

Whatever happens, I am going to be happy because I want to be. It is a choice that I recently made. I am compelling myself to be happy, but sometimes things fall apart. Things that bend me are the smallest things (no more for me) as I see both sides of the coin, seeing the danger involved in walking, talking and everyday tasks.

If I wish to change something, I will work for it rather than cribbing about it in my notepad. I cannot really change people's point of view, unless I change to be happy and positive, being content with what is and working for more.

To be reluctant as well as secure is judgment made after calculating the risk involved but, being intimidated by the fear of failure without trying and postponing something you desire are two sides of the same coin; the latter is all about being lazy. Let the horses loose if you crave betterment, but prevent them from galloping and keep the saddle in your control.

You are the manger of your happiness. It's very true that it's easier to be happy if you have perfection and basic fitness but with TBI you cannot blame yourself for your limitations: innate organs were harmed, and their regeneration has had to start all over again from level zero or they're dead and replaced by other cells.

Happiness and laughter are of course related, but happiness is intrinsic and laughter is momentary. I guess happiness comes with participation whereas laughter is like earthquake jolts, rare. I am trying on the happiness part but a few impediments are restricting it, which only strain me.

Happiness is an expensive gift that one should not expect from anyone else other than selfthemselves. It must be retrieved from within although it grows when you socialize with likeminded people. It is the juice of life which sprinkles one's mind and soul. Happiness is like a blush, a sweet, self-sustaining feeling which makes you feel lively and fresh. If you are willing to grow and improve, you must keep it in your back pack and frequently wear or carry it. There will be times when you feel nothing but pain, embarrassment and humiliation.

It's during those times that you must ask yourself, "From where did I start? What did I have? How bright were my prospects?" At that point, remember the back pack and use it. You might feel everything is destroyed and finished but it's all about not giving up.

I wrote all this but I am seriously not happy. Nothing is happening in my life to keep me happy and positive. Everyone has an advice, not because they are perfect but because from their point of view they are perfect and they think I am not trying to help myself. Every second I remind myself to be happy but I am not because I am expecting a lot from others, expecting them to understand and allow me to sync in. But they see me as an injured person and their behaviour is intolerable which make me drown. Still, amongst all of this I am positive as it helps me to flourish. I am happy with my phone notepad; it allows to me express my feelings without questions or advice, gives me time to correct myself and doesn't give a damn about other phones' notepads (unlike people).

Other people's expectations are burdensome. No one gets hurt more than me when I fail or struggle while speaking or doing the various things I do or wish to do. No one expects more from me than me, and yet still I fail to employ my methods and tricks to flourish. All of this is sucking the life out of me, making me stress more on my weak points (which are many) and stopping me from concentrating on recovery.

Irrespective of this I'm trying to be happy as stress is what bothers me and makes me sad. Perspective towards matters like stress is real whereas happiness is a choice of mind.

I often console myself by believing that this injury is temporary but one cannot change the mind-set. There was a time in my life when I struggled for acceptance but now I am settled to an extent and wish for no compensation in behaviour and treatment. I'm happy considering my journey to some extent and want to add more to it to make myself content with my situation. Stepping beyond grievances, I do not wish to change others' comfort zones; I simply want self-acceptance. My happiness is within my reach and control and doesn't require much effort other than being myself.

The good things to be happy about are short but I like them and embrace them. I have learned to do things slowly and nicely (at least I think so) and to do them without error (again, I think so). I speak slowly, which I have not done before and I like it as people understand in a single go. Most importantly I feel good about it. (Of course, if I go too slowly it becomes robotic).)

I have seen colours that are beautiful and vibrant, in flowers and on walls and clothes, but it's a fact that colours fade away after long and deep use, no matter how much you spend on them. Your spirit is something similar but it's within you, constantly pumping, asking for joy, excitement, self-motivation and self-acceptance to keep it prospering, alive and lasting.

If you're happy, you hear the voice of the spirit in your mind and within your heart. It's something you own as it's organic, and you can control and command it. When it's out of control it's easier to be depressed or crestfallen, but it takes effort to smile and be joyful.

When you feel you have always been victorious and a winner, it's tough when the situation differs. Being a winner against an opponent is a competition. Now, however, you're standing against your own gut. It's a tough competitor and it can defeat you from within, but you must not give up. Keep defending yourself and never ever surrender, as it ignites the flame in you. You might feel you're drowning, but your spirit keeps you afloat. It might be slow, but it gets you to the shore.

From all these years of suffering and pain, grief and silent happiness I have realised that no one is happy, whether he or she is struggling for a better life or is stressing over how to extract more out of it. We are further driven towards pain by the thoughts our conscious minds create. I wish to be happy or merry for the present, not neglecting my weaknesses, but working hard and making them less prominent, focussing to achieve more. Currently, happiness is my goal, and being patient despite all I have lost; I will still try to achieve what is manageable and within prescribed limits.

I am fortunate and thankful for getting another chance at the complete recovery. I see it as more of a makeover (from within) trying to get rid of toxins. I am thankful for never giving up, despite of all the depression and negativity my conscious mind creates. I have seen cases of people I knew who went from being comatose straight to the death pile. At least I could rewrite my story my way. I want to improve - foremost for my honour, and secondly to motivate others to not let vulnerability affect them in any way. The depression that everyone is dealing with might be due to a slow pace in recovery which was fast initially. I want them to trust their consciences and uplift themselves from all the grief, sorrow, expectation and depression their unconscious mind creates, hence propelling them to trust their instinct which silently says 'never give up'.

My vulnerability and my actions create a gloomy ambience which leads to hypertension. I wish to be happy and think less (about anything that doesn't remind me of my weakness). I wish I could relieve myself of negativity and concentrate more on positives, but the human brain neglects positives. As the sun dims and darkness approaches, my positivity shrinks but certain parts of my brain make way for nicer thoughts. As self confidence and trust grows, I believe this negativity must fade away.

When I complain about things, I feel that TBI has made me an escapist. It has become so difficult to be happy as I am incapable of many things. I crave happiness but it feels like happiness is running away from me and is saying, "Maintain a fair distance from me."

There are two kinds of thought processes: one elevates the good in you and the other unintentionally weighs you down, crushing the confidence and positivity present inside. It's for you to decide which of the thoughts make their way to your heart and affects you.

When people were unsure if you would lead a normal life, you had the courage to go that extra distance for yourself. Listen. If you do not treat yourself formidably don't expect it from anyone else! There must be a reason behind your survival. Perhaps that reason is still unknown but you must value your existence, just like those who know it try to convince you daily how precious you are. From this day onwards, stop cursing yourself as you aren't in a position to judge yourself. And until you can find what interests you or can earn you a decent wage, better to give your concentration, respect and obligation to whatever you are doing.

TBI key pointers:-

1. Don't be ashamed.

2. Give up on the frustration by adapting a means of entertaining yourself.

3. No one can and will take your pain.

4. Everything is expensive except advice and demonstration.

5. Friends vanish faster than leaves in autumn.

6. No-one could have done it better than you. PS: you are a survivor.

7. If you have faith in yourself and in whoever you trust, your circumstances will be better.

8. You are tired, frustrated and crestfallen but you are still capable of going further.

9. Be a motivator for yourself and never ever give up on yourself.

10. Focus on your present situation rather than impending dreams.

THE END